The Ultimate Diabetic Cookbook for Beginners

*Delicious and Simple Recipes to
Help Prevent and Control Diabetes Without Feeling Hungry*

Sophie Kruis

© **Copyright 2021 By Sophie Kruis - All rights reserved.**

The content contained within this book may not be reproduced, duplicated or transmitted without direct written permission from the author or the publisher.

Under no circumstances will any blame or legal responsibility be held against the publisher, or author, for any damages, reparation, or monetary loss due to the information contained within this book. Either directly or indirectly.

Legal Notice:

This book is copyright protected. This book is only for personal use. You cannot amend, distribute, sell, use, quote or paraphrase any part, or the content within this book, without the consent of the author or publisher.

Disclaimer Notice:

Please note the information contained within this document is for educational and entertainment purposes only. All effort has been executed to present accurate, up to date, and reliable, complete information. No warranties of any kind are declared or implied. Readers acknowledge that the author is not engaging in the rendering of legal, financial, medical or professional advice. The content within this book has been derived from various sources. Please consult a licensed professional before attempting any techniques outlined in this book.

By reading this document, the reader agrees that under no circumstances is the author responsible for any losses, direct or indirect, which are incurred as a result of the use of information contained within this document, including, but not limited to, errors, omissions, or inaccuracies.

Table Of Contents

INTRODUCTION 6

BREAKFAST RECIPES 9
1. Healthy Baked Eggs 9
2. Quick Low-Carb Oatmeal 12
3. Tofu and Vegetable Scramble 14
4. Breakfast Smoothie Bowl with Fresh Berries 17

APPETIZER RECIPES 20
5. Beet Salad with Basil Dressing 20
6. Basic Salad with Olive Oil Dressing 22
7. Spinach & Orange Salad with Oil Drizzle 23
8. Fruit Salad with Coconut-Lime Dressing 25
9. Cranberry And Brussels Sprouts With Dressing 27
10. Parsnip, Carrot, And Kale Salad with Dressing 29
11. Tomato Toasts 31
12. Everyday Salad 33

FIRST COURSE RECIPES 35
13. Green Salad with Blackberries, Goat Cheese, and Sweet Potatoes 35
14. Three Bean and Basil Salad 37
15. Rainbow Black Bean Salad 39
16. Warm Barley and Squash Salad 41

SECOND COURSE RECIPES 44
17. Mixed Chowder 44
18. Mussels in Tomato Sauce 46
19. Citrus Salmon 48
20. Herbed Salmon 50
21. Salmon in Green Sauce 52
22. Braised Shrimp 54

SIDE DISH RECIPES 57
23. Chick Pea and Kale Dish 57
24. Zucchini Chips 59
25. Classic Blueberry Spelt Muffins 61
26. Genuine Healthy Crackers 63

27.	TORTILLA CHIPS	65
28.	PUMPKIN SPICE CRACKERS	67
29.	SPICY ROASTED NUTS	69

SOUPS & STEWS 71

30.	SPICY PEPPER SOUP	71
31.	ZOODLE WON-TON SOUP	73
32.	BROCCOLI STILTON SOUP	74
33.	LAMB STEW	75
34.	IRISH STEW	76
35.	SWEET AND SOUR SOUP	77

DESSERTS 79

36.	LEMON CUSTARD	79
37.	BAKED STUFFED PEARS	81
38.	BUTTERNUT SQUASH PIE	83
39.	COCONUT CHIA CREAM POT	86
40.	CHOCOLATE AVOCADO MOUSSE	88
41.	CHIA VANILLA COCONUT PUDDING	90
42.	SWEET TAHINI DIP WITH GINGER CINNAMON FRUIT	92
43.	COCONUT BUTTER AND CHOPPED BERRIES WITH MINT	94

JUICE AND SMOOTHIE RECIPES 96

44.	PINEAPPLE & CARROT SMOOTHIE	96
45.	OATS & ORANGE SMOOTHIE	98
46.	PUMPKIN SMOOTHIE	99
47.	RED VEGGIE & FRUIT SMOOTHIE	101
48.	KALE SMOOTHIE	102
49.	GREEN TOFU SMOOTHIE	104
50.	GRAPE & SWISS CHARD SMOOTHIE	106
51.	MATCHA SMOOTHIE	107

CONCLUSION 109

Introduction

Diabetes is a condition in which the body is no longer able to self-regulate blood glucose. When you eat a food that contains carbohydrates, whether it's honey, an apple or brown rice, your body breaks it down into sugar (also called glucose) during digestion. This glucose passes through the walls of the intestine into the bloodstream, which causes an increase in blood glucose (the amount of glucose circulating in the blood). In response, the pancreas secretes a hormone called insulin. Insulin's role is to lower blood sugar to normal levels. It does this by moving sugar from the blood into cells, where it is used for energy. Think of insulin as a key that unlocks cell doors. But if you have diabetes, either your body doesn't make enough insulin, or your cells don't respond to insulin. This causes blood sugar to build up in the bloodstream, resulting in high blood sugar.

A diagnosis of diabetes means your pancreas can't make enough insulin to cope, and the result is an insulin deficiency. If your body can't produce enough insulin, your blood sugar levels become elevated. Long-term high blood sugar levels can affect almost every system in the body.

Health complications can include heart disease, stroke, kidney failure, nerve damage, eye damage, and blindness. This is why it is so important to work with your health care team to find the best treatment plan for you and for you to take the lead in your plan by eating healthy, staying physically active, and losing weight if needed. People with diabetes often think they need to focus strictly on avoiding sugar or carbohydrates and neglect to consider the nutritional quality of their diet. While it is true that carbohydrates have the greatest impact on blood sugar, it is the diet as a whole that contributes to health, weight management, and blood sugar control. Strictly limiting carbohydrates found in fruits and whole grains while eating a diet high in saturated fat and sodium does not promote optimal health.

Focusing on healthy foods, controlling carbohydrate portions, and losing weight if you're overweight are the three most important things you can do to manage type 2 diabetes from a nutritional standpoint. And don't feel pressured to reach an unrealistically low weight - even losing 5-7% of your body weight can help lower your blood sugar and reduce the need for diabetes medications.

Breakfast Recipes

1. Healthy Baked Eggs

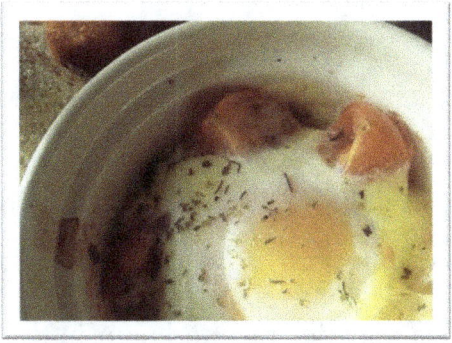

Preparation Time: 10 minutes

Cooking Time: 1 hour

Servings: 6

Ingredients:

- Olive oil – 1 tablespoon
- Garlic – 2 cloves
- Eggs – 8 larges
- Sea salt – 1/2 teaspoon
- Shredded mozzarella cheese (medium-fat) – 3 cups
- Olive oil spray
- Onion (chopped) – 1 medium

- Spinach leaves – 8 ounces
- Half-and-half – 1 cup
- Black pepper – 1 teaspoon
- Feta cheese – 1/2 cup

Directions:

1. Begin by heating the oven to 375F.
2. Get a glass baking dish and grease it with olive oil spray. Arrange aside.
3. Now take a nonstick pan and pour in the olive oil. Position the pan on allows heat and allows it heat.
4. Immediately you are done, toss in the garlic, spinach, and onion. Prepare for about 5 minutes. Arrange aside.
5. You can now Get a large mixing bowl and add in the half, eggs, pepper, and salt. Whisk thoroughly to combine.
6. Put in the feta cheese and chopped mozzarella cheese (reserve 1/2 cup of mozzarella cheese for later).
7. Put the egg mixture and prepared spinach to the prepared glass baking dish. Blend well to combine. Drizzle the reserved cheese over the top.
8. Bake the egg mix for about 45 minutes.

9. Extract the baking dish from the oven and allow it to stand for 10 minutes.

10. Dice and serve!

Nutrition: Calories: 323 calories per serving; Fat – 22.3 g; Protein – 22.6 g; Carbohydrates – 7.9 g

2. Quick Low-Carb Oatmeal

Preparation Time: 10 minutes
Cooking Time: 15 minutes
Servings: 2
Ingredients:

- Almond flour – 1/2 cup
- Flax meal – 2 tablespoons
- Cinnamon (ground) – 1 teaspoon
- Almond milk (unsweetened) – 1 1/2 cups
- Salt – as per taste
- Chia seeds – 2 tablespoons
- Liquid stevia – 10 – 15 drops
- Vanilla extract – 1 teaspoon

Directions:

1. Begin by taking a large mixing bowl and adding in the coconut flour, almond flour, ground cinnamon, flax seed powder, and chia seeds. Mix properly to combine.

2. Position a stockpot on a low heat and add in the dry ingredients. Also add in the liquid stevia, vanilla extract, and almond milk. Mix well to combine.

3. Prepare the flour and almond milk for about 4 minutes. Add salt if needed.

4. Move the oatmeal to a serving bowl and top with nuts, seeds, and pure and neat berries.

Nutrition: Calories: calories per serving; Protein – 11.7 g; Fat – 24.3 g; Carbohydrates – 16.7 g

3. Tofu and Vegetable Scramble

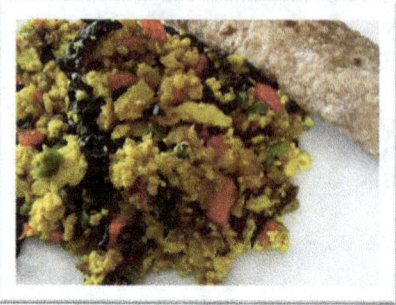

Preparation Time: 10 minutes

Cooking Time: 15 minutes

Servings: 2

Ingredients:

- Firm tofu (drained) – 16 ounces
- Sea salt – 1/2 teaspoon
- Garlic powder – 1 teaspoon
- Fresh coriander – for garnishing
- Red onion – 1/2 medium
- Cumin powder – 1 teaspoon
- Lemon juice – for topping
- Green bell pepper – 1 medium
- Garlic powder – 1 teaspoon
- Fresh coriander – for garnishing

- Red onion – 1/2 medium
- Cumin powder – 1 teaspoon
- Lemon juice – for topping

Directions:
1. Begin by preparing the ingredients. For this, you are to extract the seeds of the tomato and green bell pepper. Shred the onion, bell pepper, and tomato into small cubes.
2. Get a small mixing bowl and position the fairly hard tofu inside it. Make use of your hands to break the fairly hard tofu. Arrange aside.
3. Get a nonstick pan and add in the onion, tomato, and bell pepper. Mix and cook for about 3 minutes.
4. Put the somewhat hard crumbled tofu to the pan and combine well.
5. Get a small bowl and put in the water, turmeric, garlic powder, cumin powder, and chili powder. Combine well and stream it over the tofu and vegetable mixture.
6. Allow the tofu and vegetable crumble cook with seasoning for 5 minutes. Continuously stir so that the pan is not holding the ingredients.
7. Drizzle the tofu scramble with chili flakes and salt. Combine well.
8. Transfer the prepared scramble to a serving bowl and give it a proper spray of lemon juice.

9. Finalize by garnishing with pure and neat coriander. Serve while hot!

Nutrition: Calories: 238 calories per serving; Carbohydrates – 16.6 g; Fat – 11 g

4. Breakfast Smoothie Bowl with Fresh Berries

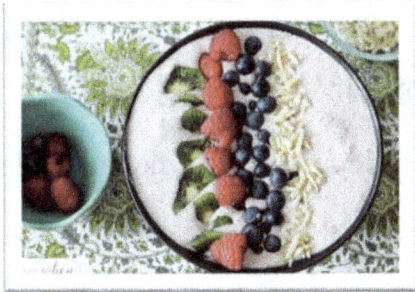

Preparation Time: 10 minutes

Cooking Time: 5 minutes

Servings: 2

Ingredients:

- Almond milk (unsweetened) – 1/2 cup
- Psyllium husk powder – 1/2 teaspoon
- Strawberries (chopped) – 2 ounces
- Coconut oil – 1 tablespoon
- Crushed ice – 3 cups
- Liquid stevia – 5 to 10 drops
- Pea protein powder – 1/3 cup

Directions:

1. Begin by taking a blender and adding in the mashed ice cubes. Allow them to rest for about 30 seconds.

2. Then put in the almond milk, shredded strawberries, pea protein powder, psyllium husk powder, coconut oil, and liquid stevia. Blend well until it turns into a smooth and creamy puree.

3. Vacant the prepared smoothie into 2 glasses.

4. Cover with coconut flakes and pure and neat strawberries.

Nutrition: Calories: 166 calories per serving; Fat – 9.2 g; Carbohydrates – 4.1 g; Protein – 17.6 g

Appetizer Recipes

5. Beet Salad with Basil Dressing

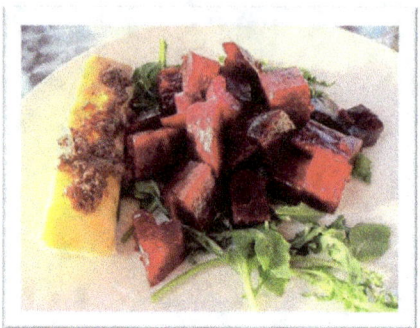

Preparation Time: 10 minutes

Cooking Time: 0 minutes

Servings: 4

Ingredients:

Ingredients for the dressing

- ¼ cup blackberries
- ¼ cup extra-virgin olive oil
- Juice of 1 lemon
- 2 tablespoons minced fresh basil
- 1 teaspoon poppy seeds
- A pinch of sea salt
- For the salad

- 2 celery stalks, chopped
- 4 cooked beets, peeled and chopped
- 1 cup blackberries
- 4 cups spring mix

Directions:
1. To make the dressing, mash the blackberries in a bowl. Whisk in the oil, lemon juice, basil, poppy seeds, and sea salt.
2. To make the salad: Add the celery, beets, blackberries, and spring mix to the bowl with the dressing.
3. Combine and serve.

Nutrition: Calories: 192; Fat: 15g; Carbohydrates: 15g; Protein: 2g

6. Basic Salad with Olive Oil Dressing

Preparation Time: 10 minutes

Cooking Time: 0 minute

Servings: 4

Ingredients:

- 1 cup coarsely chopped iceberg lettuce
- 1 cup coarsely chopped romaine lettuce
- 1 cup fresh baby spinach
- 1 large tomato, hulled and coarsely chopped
- 1 cup diced cucumber
- 2 tablespoons extra-virgin olive oil
- ¼ teaspoon of sea salt

Directions:

1. In a bowl, combine the spinach and lettuces. Add the tomato and cucumber.
2. Drizzle with oil and sprinkle with sea salt.
3. Mix and serve.

Nutrition: Calories: 77; Fat: 4g; Carbohydrates: 3g; Protein: 1g

7. Spinach & Orange Salad with Oil Drizzle

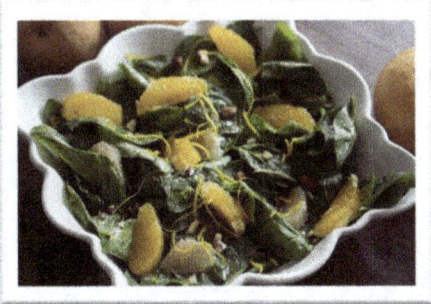

Preparation Time: 10 minutes

Cooking Time: 0 minute

Servings: 4

Ingredients:

- 4 cups fresh baby spinach
- 1 blood orange, coarsely chopped
- ½ red onion, thinly sliced
- ½ shallot, finely chopped
- 2 tbsp. minced fennel fronds
- Juice of 1 lemon
- 1 tbsp. extra-virgin olive oil
- Pinch sea salt

Directions:

1. In a bowl, toss together the spinach, orange, red onion, shallot, and fennel fronds.

2. Add the lemon juice, oil, and sea salt.

3. Mix and serve.

Nutrition: Calories: 79; Fat: 2g; Carbohydrates: 8g; Protein: 1g

8. Fruit Salad with Coconut-Lime Dressing

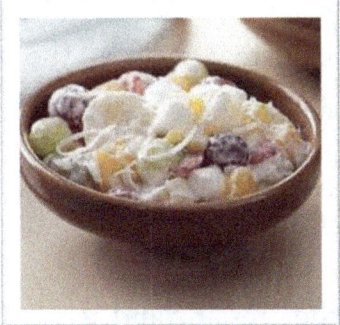

Preparation Time: 5 minutes

Cooking Time: 0 minutes

Servings: 4

Ingredients:

Ingredients for the dressing

- ¼ cup full-fat canned coconut milk
- 1 tbsp. raw honey
- Juice of ½ lime
- Pinch sea salt
- For the salad
- 2 bananas, thinly sliced
- 2 mandarin oranges, segmented
- ½ cup strawberries, thinly sliced
- ½ cup raspberries

- ½ cup blueberries

Directions:

1. To make the dressing: whisk all the dressing Ingredients in a bowl.

2. To make the salad: Add the salad Ingredients in a bowl and mix.

3. Drizzle with the dressing and serve.

Nutrition: Calories: 141; Fat: 3g; Carbohydrates: 30g; Protein: 2g

9. Cranberry And Brussels Sprouts With Dressing

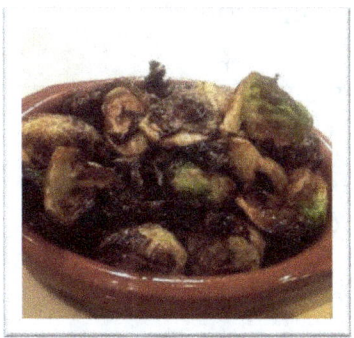

Preparation Time: 10 minutes

Cooking Time: 0 minute

Servings: 4

Ingredients:

Ingredients for the dressing

- 1/3 cup extra-virgin olive oil
- 2 tbsp. apple cider vinegar
- 1 tbsp. pure maple syrup
- Juice of 1 orange
- ½ tbsp. dried rosemary
- 1 tbsp. scallion, whites only
- Pinch sea salt

For the salad

- 1 bunch scallions, greens only, finely chopped

- 1 cup Brussels sprouts, stemmed, halved, and thinly sliced
- ½ cup fresh cranberries
- 4 cups fresh baby spinach

Directions:

1. To make the dressing: In a bowl, whisk the dressing Ingredients.
2. To make the salad: Add the scallions, Brussels sprouts, cranberries, and spinach to the bowl with the dressing.
3. Combine and serve.

Nutrition: Calories: 267; Fat: 18g; Carbohydrates: 26g; Protein: 2g

10. Parsnip, Carrot, And Kale Salad with Dressing

Preparation Time: 10 minutes
Cooking Time: 0 minutes
Servings: 4
Ingredients:
Ingredients for the dressing

- 1/3 cup extra-virgin olive oil
- Juice of 1 lime
- 2 tbsp. minced fresh mint leaves
- 1 tsp. pure maple syrup
- Pinch sea salt

For the salad

- 1 bunch kale, chopped
- ½ parsnip, grated
- ½ carrot, grated
- 2 tbsp. sesame seeds

Directions:

1. To make the dressing, mix all the dressing Ingredients in a bowl.

2. To make the salad, add the kale to the dressing and massage the dressing into the kale for 1 minute.

3. Add the parsnip, carrot, and sesame seeds.

4. Combine and serve.

Nutrition: Calories: 214; Fat: 2g; Carbohydrates: 12g; Protein: 2g

11. Tomato Toasts

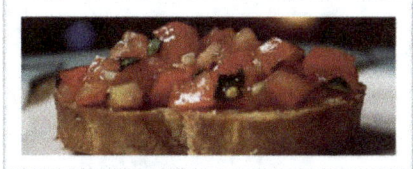

Preparation Time: 5 minutes

Cooking Time: 5 minutes

Servings: 4

Ingredients:

- 4 slices of sprouted bread toasts
- 2 tomatoes, sliced
- 1 avocado, mashed
- 1 teaspoon olive oil
- 1 pinch of salt
- ¾ teaspoon ground black pepper

Directions:

1. Blend together the olive oil, mashed avocado, salt, and ground black pepper.
2. When the mixture is homogenous – spread it over the sprouted bread.
3. Then place the sliced tomatoes over the toasts.
4. Enjoy!

Nutrition: Calories: 125; Fat: 11.1g; Carbohydrates: 7.0g; Protein: 1.5g

12. Everyday Salad

Preparation Time: 10 minutes
Cooking Time: 40 minutes
Servings: 6
Ingredients:

- 5 halved mushrooms
- 6 halved Cherry (Plum) Tomatoes
- 6 rinsed Lettuce Leaves
- 10 olives
- ½ chopped cucumber
- Juice from ½ Key Lime
- 1 teaspoon olive oil
- Pure Sea Salt

Directions:

1. Tear rinsed lettuce leaves into medium pieces and put them in a medium salad bowl.
2. Add mushrooms halves, chopped cucumber, olives and cherry tomato halves into the bowl. Mix well. Pour olive and Key Lime juice over salad.
3. Add pure sea salt to taste. Mix it all till it is well combined.

Nutrition: Calories: 88; Carbohydrates: 11g; Fat: 5g; Protein: 8g

First Course Recipes

13. Green Salad with Blackberries, Goat Cheese, and Sweet Potatoes

Preparation Time: 15 minutes

Cooking Time: 20 minutes

Serving: 4

Ingredients:

For the vinaigrette

- 1-pint blackberries
- 2 tablespoons red wine vinegar
- 1 tablespoon honey
- 3 tablespoons extra-virgin olive oil
- ¼ teaspoon salt
- Freshly ground black pepper

For the salad

- 1 sweet potato, cubed
- 1 teaspoon extra-virgin olive oil
- 8 cups salad greens (baby spinach, spicy greens, romaine)
- ½ red onion, sliced

- ¼ cup crumbled goat cheese

Directions:

For vinaigrette

1. In a blender jar, combine the blackberries, vinegar, honey, oil, salt, and pepper, and process until smooth. Set aside.

For salad

2. Preheat the oven to 425°F. Line a baking sheet with parchment paper.

3. Mix the sweet potato with the olive oil. Transfer to the prepared baking sheet and roast for 20 minutes, stirring once halfway through, until tender. Remove and cool for a few minutes.

4. In a large bowl, toss the greens with the red onion and cooled sweet potato, and drizzle with the vinaigrette. Serve topped with 1 tablespoon of goat cheese per serving.

Nutrition: 196 Calories; 21g Carbohydrates; 10g Sugars

14. Three Bean and Basil Salad

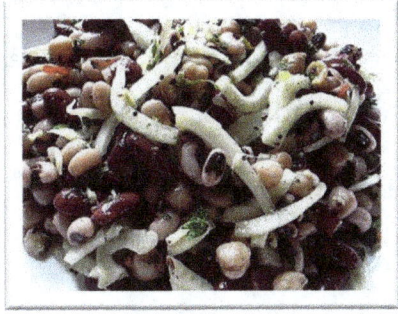

Preparation Time: 10 minutes

Cooking Time: 0 minute

Serving: 8

Ingredients:

- 1 (15-ounce) can low-sodium chickpeas
- 1 (15-ounce) can low-sodium kidney beans
- 1 (15-ounce) can low-sodium white beans
- 1 red bell pepper
- ¼ cup chopped scallions
- ¼ cup finely chopped fresh basil
- 3 garlic cloves, minced
- 2 tablespoons extra-virgin olive oil
- 1 tablespoon red wine vinegar
- 1 teaspoon Dijon mustard

- ¼ teaspoon freshly ground black pepper

Directions:
1. Toss chickpeas, kidney beans, white beans, bell pepper, scallions, basil, and garlic gently.
2. Blend together olive oil, vinegar, mustard, and pepper. Toss with the salad.
3. Wrap and chill for 1 hour.

Nutrition: 193 Calories; 29g Carbohydrates; 3g Sugars

15. Rainbow Black Bean Salad

Preparation Time: 15 minutes
Cooking Time: 0 minute
Serving: 5
Ingredients:

- 1 (15-ounce) can low-sodium black beans
- 1 avocado, diced
- 1 cup cherry
- tomatoes, halved
- 1 cup chopped baby spinach
- ½ cup red bell pepper
- ¼ cup jicama
- ½ cup scallions
- ¼ cup fresh cilantro
- 2 tablespoons lime juice
- 1 tablespoon extra-virgin olive oil
- 2 garlic cloves, minced
- 1 teaspoon honey
- ¼ teaspoon salt

- ¼ teaspoon freshly ground black pepper

Directions:
1. Mix black beans, avocado, tomatoes, spinach, bell pepper, jicama, scallions, and cilantro.
2. Blend lime juice, oil, garlic, honey, salt, and pepper. Add to the salad and toss.
3. Chill for 1 hour before serving.

Nutrition: 169 Calories; 22g Carbohydrates; 3g Sugars

16. Warm Barley and Squash Salad

Preparation Time: 20 minutes
Cooking Time: 40 minutes
Serving: 8
Ingredients:

- 1 small butternut squash
- 3 tablespoons extra-virgin olive oil
- 2 cups broccoli florets
- 1 cup pearl barley
- 1 cup toasted chopped walnuts
- 2 cups baby kale
- ½ red onion, sliced
- 2 tablespoons balsamic vinegar
- 2 garlic cloves, minced
- ½ teaspoon salt
- ¼ teaspoon black pepper

Directions:
1. Preheat the oven to 400°F. Line a baking sheet with parchment paper.

2. Peel off the squash, and slice into dice. In a large bowl, toss the squash with 2 teaspoons of olive oil. Transfer to the prepared baking sheet and roast for 20 minutes.

3. While the squash is roasting, toss the broccoli in the same bowl with 1 teaspoon of olive oil. After 20 minutes, flip the squash and push it to one side of the baking sheet. Add the broccoli to the other side and continue to roast for 20 more minutes until tender.

4. While the veggies are roasting, in a medium pot, cover the barley with several inches of water. Boil, then adjust heat, cover, and simmer for 30 minutes until tender. Drain and rinse.

5. Transfer the barley to a large bowl, and toss with the cooked squash and broccoli, walnuts, kale, and onion.

6. In a small bowl, mix the remaining 2 tablespoons of olive oil, balsamic vinegar, garlic, salt, and pepper. Drizzle dressing over the salad and toss.

Nutrition: 274 Calories; 32g Carbohydrates; 3g Sugars

Second Course Recipes

17. Mixed Chowder

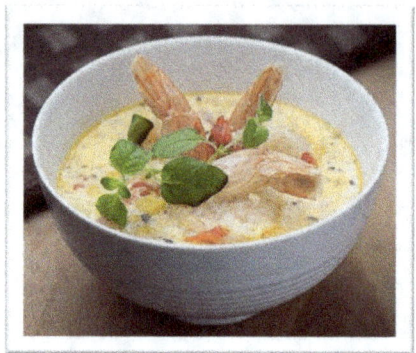

Preparation Time: 10 minutes

Cooking Time: 35 Minutes

Servings: 2

Ingredients:
- 1lb fish stew mix
- 2 cups white sauce
- 3tbsp old bay seasoning

Directions:
1. Mix all the ingredients in your Instant Pot.
2. Cook on Stew for 35 minutes.
3. Release the pressure naturally.

Nutrition: Calories: 320; Carbs: 9; Sugar: 2; Fat: 16; Protein: GL: 4

18. Mussels in Tomato Sauce

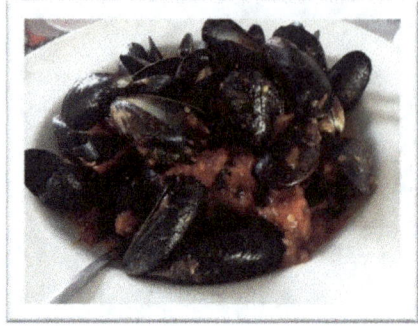

Preparation Time: 10 minutes

Cooking Time: 3 Minutes

Servings: 4

Ingredients:

- 2 tomatoes, seeded and chopped finely
- 2 pounds mussels, scrubbed and de-bearded
- 1 cup low-sodium chicken broth
- 1 tablespoon fresh lemon juice
- 2 garlic cloves, minced

Directions:

1. In the pot of Instant Pot, place tomatoes, garlic, wine and bay leaf and stir to combine.
2. Arrange the mussels on top.
3. Close the lid and place the pressure valve to "Seal" position.

4. Press "Manual" and cook under "High Pressure" for about 3 minutes.

5. Press "Cancel" and carefully allow a "Quick" release.

6. Open the lid and serve hot.

Nutrition: Calories: 213; Fats: 25.2g; Carbs: 11g; Sugar: 1; Proteins: 28.2g; Sodium: 670mg

19. Citrus Salmon

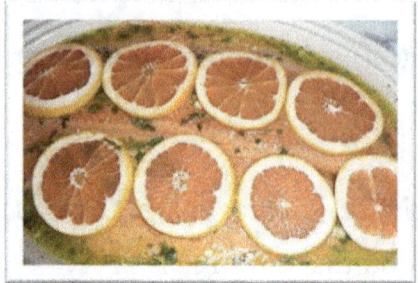

Preparation Time: 10 minutes

Cooking Time: 7 Minutes

Servings: 4

Ingredients:

- 4 (4-ounce) salmon fillets
- 1 cup low-sodium chicken broth
- 1 teaspoon fresh ginger, minced
- 2 teaspoons fresh orange zest, grated finely
- 3 tablespoons fresh orange juice
- 1 tablespoon olive oil
- Ground black pepper, as required

Directions:

1. In Instant Pot, add all ingredients and mix.
2. Close the lid and place the pressure valve to "Seal" position.

3. Press "Manual" and cook under "High Pressure" for about 7 minutes.

4. Press "Cancel" and allow a "Natural" release.

5. Open the lid and serve the salmon fillets with the topping of cooking sauce.

Nutrition: Calories: 190; Fats: 10.5g; Carbs: 1.8g; Sugar: 1g; Proteins: 22. Sodium: 68mg

20. Herbed Salmon

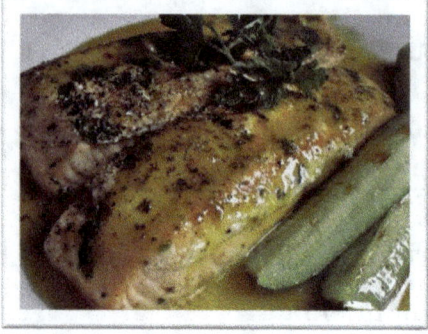

Preparation Time: 10 minutes
Cooking Time: 3 Minutes
Servings: 4
Ingredients:

- 4 (4-ounce) salmon fillets
- ¼ cup olive oil
- 2 tablespoons fresh lemon juice
- 1 garlic clove, minced
- ¼ teaspoon dried oregano
- Salt and ground black pepper, as required
- 4 fresh rosemary sprigs
- 4 lemon slices

Directions:

1. For dressing: in a large bowl, add oil, lemon juice, garlic, oregano, salt and black pepper and beat until well co combined.

2. Arrange a steamer trivet in the Instant Pot and pour 1 1/2 cups of water in Instant Pot.

3. Place the salmon fillets on top of trivet in a single layer and top with dressing.

4. Arrange 1 rosemary sprig and 1 lemon slice over each fillet.

5. Close the lid and place the pressure valve to "Seal" position.

6. Press "Steam" and just use the default time of 3 minutes.

7. Press "Cancel" and carefully allow a "Quick" release.

8. Open the lid and serve hot.

Nutrition: Calories: 262; Fats: 17g; Carbs: 0.7g; Sugar: 0.2g; Proteins: 22.1g; Sodium: 91mg

21. Salmon in Green Sauce

Preparation Time: 10 minutes

Cooking Time: 12 Minutes

Servings: 4

Ingredients:

- 4 (6-ounce) salmon fillets
- 1 avocado, peeled, pitted and chopped
- 1/2 cup fresh basil, chopped
- 3 garlic cloves, chopped
- 1 tablespoon fresh lemon zest, grated finely

Directions:

1. Grease a large piece of foil.
2. In a large bowl, add all ingredients except salmon and water and with a fork, mash completely.
3. Place fillets in the center of foil and top with avocado mixture evenly.
4. Fold the foil around fillets to seal them.
5. Arrange a steamer trivet in the Instant Pot and pour 1/2 cup of water.
6. Place the foil packet on top of trivet.

7. Close the lid and place the pressure valve to "Seal" position.

8. Press "Manual" and cook under "High Pressure" for about minutes.

9. Meanwhile, preheat the oven to broiler.

10. Press "Cancel" and allow a "Natural" release.

11. Open the lid and transfer the salmon fillets onto a broiler pan.

12. Broil for about 3-4 minutes.

13. Serve warm.

Nutrition: Calories: 333; Fats: 20.3g; Carbs: 5.5g; Sugar: 0.4g; Proteins; 34.2g; Sodium: 79mg

22. Braised Shrimp

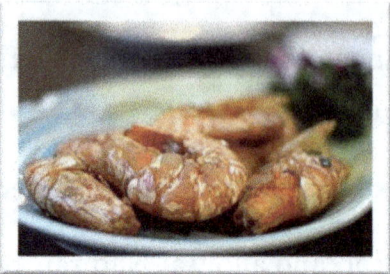

Preparation Time: 10 minutes

Cooking Time: 4 Minutes

Servings: 4

Ingredients:

- 1-pound frozen large shrimp, peeled and deveined
- 2 shallots, chopped
- ¾ cup low-sodium chicken broth
- 2 tablespoons fresh lemon juice
- 2 tablespoons olive oil
- 1 tablespoon garlic, crushed
- Ground black pepper, as required

Directions:

1. In the Instant Pot, place oil and press "Sauté". Now add the shallots and cook for about 2 minutes.
2. Add the garlic and cook for about 1 minute.

3. Press "Cancel" and stir in the shrimp, broth, lemon juice and black pepper.

4. Close the lid and place the pressure valve to "Seal" position.

5. Press "Manual" and cook under "High Pressure" for about 1 minute.

6. Press "Cancel" and carefully allow a "Quick" release.

7. Open the lid and serve hot.

Nutrition: Calories: 209; Fats: 9g; Carbs: 4.3g; Sugar: 0.2g; Proteins: 26.6g; Sodium: 293mg

Side Dish Recipes

23. Chick Pea and Kale Dish

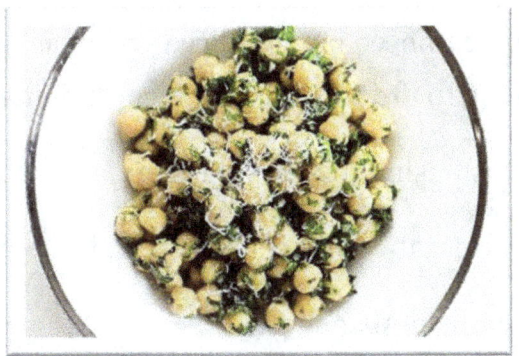

Preparation Time: 10 minutes

Cooking Time: 25-30 minutes

Servings:4

Ingredients:

- 2 cups chickpea flour
- 1/2 cup green bell pepper, diced
- 1/2 cup onions, minced
- 1 tablespoon oregano
- 1 tablespoon salt
- 1 teaspoon cayenne
- 4 cups spring water

- 2 tablespoons Grape Seed Oil

Directions:

1. Boil spring water in a large pot
2. Lower heat into medium and whisk in chickpea flour
3. Add some minced onions, diced green bell pepper, seasoning to the pot and cook for 10 minutes
4. Cover dish using a baking sheet, grease with oil
5. Pour batter into the sheet and spread with a spatula
6. Cover with another sheet
7. Transfer to a fridge and chill, for 20 minutes
8. Remove from freezer and cut batter into fry shapes
9. Preheat the Air Fryer, to 385 degrees F
10. Transfer fries into the cooking basket, lightly greased and cover with parchment
11. Bake for about 15 minutes, flip and bake for 10 minutes more until golden brown
12. Serve and enjoy!

Nutrition: Calories: 271 kcal; Carbohydrates: 28 g; Fat: 15 g; Protein: 9 g

24. Zucchini Chips

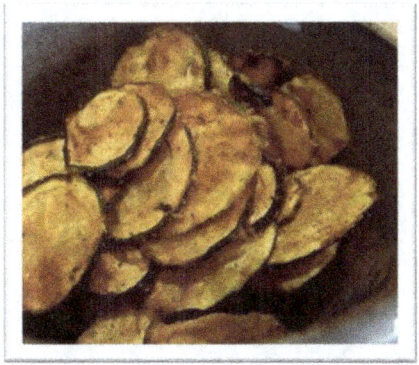

Preparation Time: 10 minutes
Cooking Time: 12-15 minutes
Servings: 4
Ingredients:

- Salt as needed
- Grape seed oil as needed
- 6 zucchinis

Directions:

1. Into 330 F, pre heat the Air Fryer
2. Wash zucchini, slice zucchini into thin strips
3. Put slices in a bowl and add oil, salt, and toss
4. Spread over the cooking basket, fry for 12-15 minutes
5. Serve and enjoy!

Nutrition: Calories: 92 kcal; Carbohydrates: 6 g; Fat: 7 g; Protein: 2 g

25. Classic Blueberry Spelt Muffins

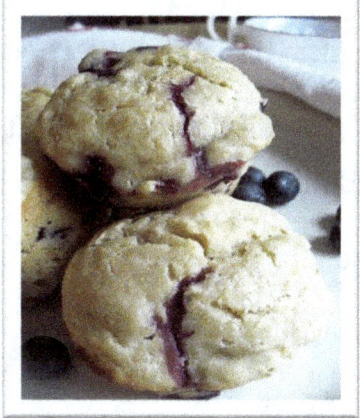

Preparation Time: 10 minutes

Cooking Time: 12-15 minutes

Servings:4

Ingredients:

- 1/4 sea salt

- 1/3 cup maple syrup

- 1 teaspoon baking powder

- 1/2 cup sea moss

- 3/4 cup spelt flour

- 3/4 cup Kamut flour

- 1 cup hemp milk

- 1 cup blueberries

Directions:

1. Into 380 degrees F pre heat Air Fryer

2. Take your muffin tins and gently grease them

3. Take a bowl and add flour, syrup, salt, baking powder, seamless and mix well

4. Add milk and mix well

5. Fold in blueberries

6. Pour into muffin tins

7. Transfer to the cooking basket, bake for 20-25 minutes until nicely baked

8. Serve and enjoy!

Nutrition: Calories: 217 kcal; Carbohydrates: 32 g; Fat: 9 g; Protein: 4 g

26. Genuine Healthy Crackers

Preparation Time: 10 minutes

Cooking Time: 12-15 minutes

Servings:4

Ingredients:
- 1/2 cup Rye flour
- 1 cup spelt flour
- 2 teaspoons sesame seed
- 1 teaspoon agave syrup
- 1 teaspoon salt
- 2 tablespoons grapeseed oil
- 3/4 cup spring water

Directions:
1. Into 330 degrees F, Preheat the Air Fryer
2. Take a medium bowl and add all Ingredients, mix well
3. Make dough ball
4. Prepare a place for rolling out the dough, cover with a piece of parchment
5. Lightly grease paper with grape seed oil, place dough
6. Roll out, dough with a rolling pin, add more flour if needed

7. Take a shape cutter and cut dough into squares

8. Place squares in Air Fryer cooking basket

9. Brush with more oil

10. Sprinkle salt

11. Bake for 10-15 minutes until golden

12. Let it cool, serve, and enjoy!

Nutrition: Calories: 226 kcal; Carbohydrates: 41 g; Fat: 3 g; Protein: 11 g

27. Tortilla Chips

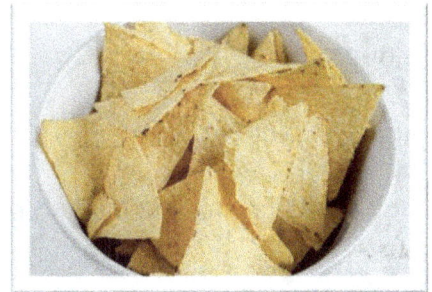

Preparation Time: 10 minutes

Cooking Time: 8-12 minutes

Servings: 4

Ingredients:

- 2 cups of spelt flour
- 1 teaspoon of salt
- 1/2 cup of spring water
- 1/3 cup of grapeseed oil

Directions:

1. Preheat your Air Fryer into 320 degrees F
2. Take the food processor then add salt, flour, and process well for 15 seconds
3. Gradually add grapeseed oil until mixed
4. Keep mixing until you have a nice dough

5. Formulate work surface and cover in a piece of parchment, sprinkle flour

6. Knead the dough for 1-2 minutes

7. Grease cooking basket with oil

8. Transfer dough on the cooking basket, brush oil and sprinkle salt

9. Cut dough into 8 triangles

10. Bake for about 8-12 minutes until golden brown

11. Serve and enjoy once done!

Nutrition: Calories: 288 kcal; Carbohydrates: 18 g; Fat: 17 g; Protein: 16 g

28. Pumpkin Spice Crackers

Preparation Time: 10 minutes
Cooking Time: 60 minutes
Servings: 6
Ingredients:
- 1/3 cup coconut flour
- 2 tablespoons pumpkin pie spice
- ¾ cup sunflower seeds
- ¾ cup flaxseed
- 1/3 cup sesame seeds
- 1 tablespoon ground psyllium husk powder
- 1 teaspoon sea salt
- 3 tablespoons coconut oil, melted
- 1 1/3 cups alkaline water

Directions:
1. Set your oven to 300 degrees F.
2. Combine all dry Ingredients in a bowl.
3. Add water and oil to the mixture and mix well.
4. Let the dough stay for 2 to 3 minutes.

5. Spread the dough evenly on a cookie sheet lined with parchment paper.

6. Bake for 30 minutes.

7. Reduce the oven heat to low and bake for another 30 minutes.

8. Crack the bread into bite-size pieces.

9. Serve

Nutrition: Calories 248; Total Fat 15.7 g; Saturated Fat 2.7 g; Cholesterol 75 mg; Sodium 94 mg; Total Carbs 0.4 g; Fiber 0g; Sugar 0 g; Protein 24.9 g

29. Spicy Roasted Nuts

Preparation Time: 10 minutes

Cooking Time: 15 minutes

Servings: 4

Ingredients:

- 8 oz. pecans or almonds or walnuts
- 1 teaspoon sea salt
- 1 tablespoon olive oil or coconut oil
- 1 teaspoon ground cumin
- 1 teaspoon paprika powder or chili powder

Directions:

1. Add all the Ingredients to a skillet.
2. Roast the nuts until golden brown.
3. Serve and enjoy.

Nutrition: Calories 287; Total Fat 29.5 g; Saturated Fat 3 g; Cholesterol 0 mg; Total Carbs 5.9 g; Sugar 1.4g; Fiber 4.3 g; Sodium 388 mg; Protein 4.2 g

Soups & Stews

30. Spicy Pepper Soup

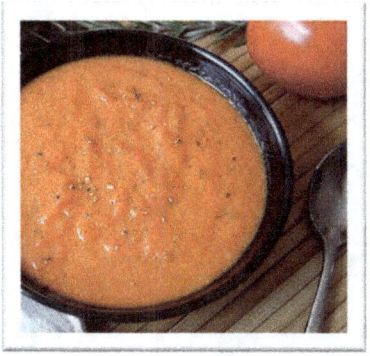

Preparation Time: 15 minutes

Cooking Time: 15 minutes

Servings: 2

Ingredients:

- 1lb chopped mixed sweet peppers
- 1 cup low sodium vegetable broth
- 3tbsp chopped chili peppers
- 1tbsp black pepper

Recipe:

1. Mix all the ingredients in your Instant Pot.
2. Cook on Stew for 15 minutes.
3. Release the pressure naturally. Blend.

Nutrition: Calories: 100; Carbs: 11; Sugar: 4; Fat: 2; Protein: 3; GL: 6

31. Zoodle Won-Ton Soup

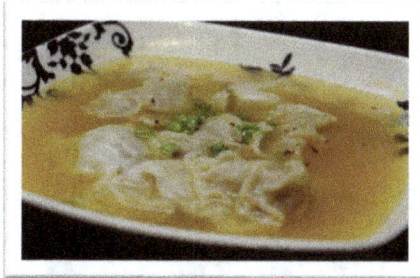

Preparation Time: 15 minutes

Cooking Time: 5 minutes

Servings: 2

Ingredients:

- 1lb spiralized zucchini
- 1 pack unfried won-tons
- 1 cup low sodium beef broth
- 2tbsp soy sauce

Recipe:

1. Mix all the ingredients in your Instant Pot.
2. Cook on Stew for 5 minutes.
3. Release the pressure naturally.

Nutrition: Calories: 300; Carbs: 6; Sugar: 1; Fat: 9; Protein: 43; GL: 2

32. Broccoli Stilton Soup

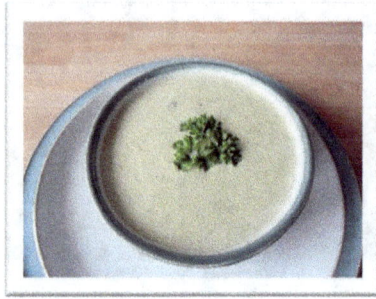

Preparation Time: 15 minutes

Cooking Time: 35 minutes

Servings: 2

Ingredients:

- 1lb chopped broccoli
- 0.5lb chopped vegetables
- 1 cup low sodium vegetable broth
- 1 cup Stilton

Recipe:

1. Mix all the ingredients in your Instant Pot.
2. Cook on Stew for 35 minutes.
3. Release the pressure naturally.
4. Blend the soup.

Nutrition: Calories: 280; Carbs: 9; Sugar: 2; Fat: 22; Protein: 13; GL: 4

33. Lamb Stew

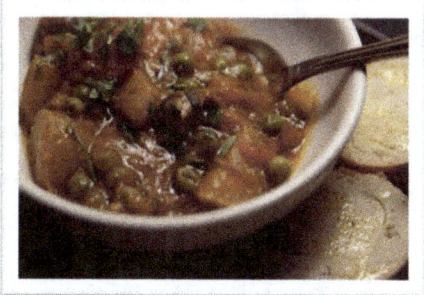

Preparation Time: 15 minutes

Cooking Time: 35 minutes

Servings: 2

Ingredients:

- 1lb diced lamb shoulder
- 1lb chopped winter vegetables
- 1 cup low sodium vegetable broth
- 1tbsp yeast extract
- 1tbsp star anise spice mix

Recipe:

1. Mix all the ingredients in your Instant Pot.
2. Cook on Stew for 35 minutes.
3. Release the pressure naturally.

Nutrition: Calories: 320; Carbs: 10; Sugar: 2; Fat: 8; Protein: 42; GL: 3

34. Irish Stew

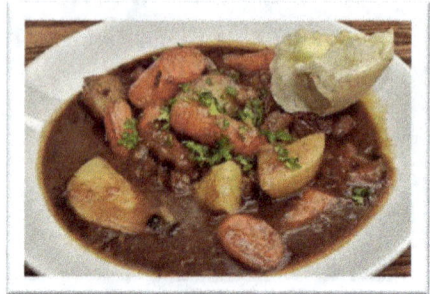

Preparation Time: 15 minutes

Cooking Time: 35 minutes

Servings: 2

Ingredients:

- 1.5lb diced lamb shoulder
- 1lb chopped vegetables
- 1 cup low sodium beef broth
- 3 minced onions
- 1tbsp ghee

Recipe:

1. Mix all the ingredients in your Instant Pot.
2. Cook on Stew for 35 minutes.
3. Release the pressure naturally.

Nutrition: Calories: 330; Carbs: 9; Sugar: 2; Fat: 12; Protein: 49; GL: 3

35. Sweet and Sour Soup

Preparation Time: 15 minutes

Cooking Time: 35 minutes

Servings: 2

Ingredients:
- 1lb cubed chicken breast
- 1lb chopped vegetables
- 1 cup low carb sweet and sour sauce
- 0.5 cup diabetic marmalade

Recipe:
1. Mix all the ingredients in your Instant Pot.
2. Cook on Stew for 35 minutes.
3. Release the pressure naturally.

Desserts

36. Lemon Custard

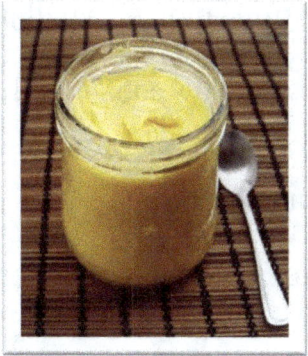

Preparation Time: 10 minutes

Cooking Time: 3 hours

Servings: 4

Ingredients:

- 2 cups whipping cream or coconut cream
- 5 egg yolks
- 1 tablespoon lemon zest
- 1 teaspoon vanilla extract
- 1/4 cup fresh lemon juice, squeezed
- 1/2 teaspoon liquid stevia
- Lightly sweetened whipped cream

Directions:

1. Whisk egg yolks together with lemon zest, liquid stevia, lemon zest and vanilla in a bowl, and then whisk in heavy cream.

2. Divide the mixture among 4 small jars or ramekins.

3. To the bottom of a slow cooker add a rack, and then add ramekins on top of the rack and add enough water to cover half of ramekins.

4. Close the lid and cook for 3 hours on low. Remove ramekins.

5. Let cool to room temperature, and then place into the refrigerator to cool completely for about 3 hours.

6. When through, top with the whipped cream and serve. Enjoy!

Nutrition: 319 Calories; 30 g Fat; 3 g Total Carbs; 7 g Protein

37. Baked Stuffed Pears

Preparation Time: 15 minutes
Cooking Time: 35 minutes
Servings: 4
Ingredients:
- Agave syrup, 4 tbsp.
- Cloves, .25 tsp.
- Chopped walnuts, 4 tbsp.
- Currants, 1 c
- Pears, 4

Directions:
1. Make sure your oven has been warmed to 375.
2. Slice the pears in two lengthwise and remove the core. To get the pear to lay flat, you can slice a small piece off the back side.
3. Place the agave syrup, currants, walnuts, and cloves in a small bowl and mix well. Set this to the side to be used later.
4. Put the pears on a cookie sheet that has parchment paper on it. Make sure the cored sides are facing up.

Sprinkle each pear half with about .5 tablespoon of the chopped walnut mixture.

5. Place into the oven and cook for 25 to 30 minutes. Pears should be tender.

Nutrition: Calories: 103.9; Fiber: 3.1 g; Carbohydrates: 22 g

38. Butternut Squash Pie

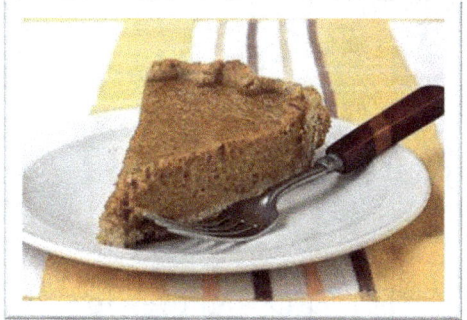

Preparation Time: 25 minutes

Cooking Time: 35 minutes

Servings: 4

Ingredients:

- For the Crust
- Cold water
- Agave, splash
- Sea salt, pinch
- Grapeseed oil, .5 c
- Coconut flour, .5 c
- Spelt Flour, 1 c
- For the Filling
- Butternut squash, peeled, chopped
- Water

- Allspice, to taste

- Agave syrup, to taste

- Hemp milk, 1 c

- Sea moss, 4 tbsp.

<u>*Directions*</u>:

1. You will need to warm your oven to 350.

2. For the Crust

3. Place the grapeseed oil and water into the refrigerator to get it cold. This will take about one hour.

4. Place all Ingredients into a large bowl. Now you need to add in the cold water a little bit in small amounts until a dough form. Place this onto a surface that has been sprinkled with some coconut flour. Knead for a few minutes and roll the dough as thin as you can get it. Carefully, pick it up and place it inside a pie plate.

5. Place the butternut squash into a Dutch oven and pour in enough water to cover. Bring this to a full rolling boil. Let this cook until the squash has become soft.

6. Completely drain and place into bowl. Using a potato masher, mash the squash. Add in some allspice and agave to taste. Add in the sea moss and hemp milk. Using a hand mixer, blend well. Pour into the pie crust.

7. Place into an oven and bake for about one hour.

Nutrition: Calories: 245; Carbohydrates: 50 g; Fat: 10 g

39. Coconut Chia Cream Pot

Preparation Time: 5 minutes
Cooking Time: 5 minutes
Servings: 4
Ingredients:

- Date, one (1)

- Coconut milk (organic), one (1) cup

- Coconut yogurt, one (1) cup

- Vanilla extract, ½ teaspoon

- Chia seeds, ¼ cup

- Sesame seeds, one (1) teaspoon

- Flaxseed (ground), one (1) tablespoon or flax meal, one (1) tablespoon

- Toppings:

- Fig, one (1)

- Blueberries, one (1) handful

- Mixed nuts (brazil nuts, almonds, pistachios, macadamia, etc.)

- Cinnamon (ground), one teaspoon

Directions:
1. First, blend the date with coconut milk (the idea is to sweeten the coconut milk).
2. Get a mixing bowl and add the coconut milk with the vanilla, sesame seeds, chia seeds, and flax meal.
3. Refrigerate for between twenty to thirty minutes or wait till the chia expands.
4. To serve, pour a layer of coconut yogurt in a small glass, then add the chia mix, followed by pouring another layer of the coconut yogurt.
5. It's alkaline, creamy and delicious.

Nutrition: Calories: 310; Carbohydrates: 39 g; Protein: 4 g; Fiber: 8.1 g

40. Chocolate Avocado Mousse

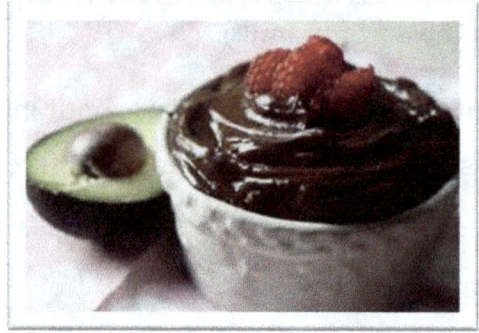

Preparation Time: 10 minutes

Cooking Time: 5 minutes

Servings: 4

Ingredients:

- Coconut water, 2/3 cup
- Avocado, ½ hass
- Raw cacao, 2 teaspoons
- Vanilla, 1 teaspoon
- Dates, three (3)
- Sea salt, one (1) teaspoon
- Dark chocolate shavings

Directions:

1. Blend all Ingredients.
2. Blast until it becomes thick and smooth, as you wish.

3. Put in a fridge and allow it to get firm.

Nutrition: Calories: 181.8; Fat: 151. G; Protein: 12 g

41. Chia Vanilla Coconut Pudding

Preparation Time: 5 minutes
Cooking Time: 5 minutes
Servings: 2
Ingredients:

- Coconut oil, 2 tablespoons
- Raw cashew, ½ cup
- Coconut water, ½ cup
- Cinnamon, 1 teaspoon
- Dates (pitted), 3
- Vanilla, 2 teaspoons
- Coconut flakes (unsweetened), 1 teaspoon
- Salt (Himalayan or Celtic Grey)
- Chia seeds, 6 tablespoons
- Cinnamon or pomegranate seeds for garnish (optional)

Directions:

1. Get a blender, add all the Ingredients (minus the pomegranate and chia seeds), and blend for about forty to sixty seconds.
2. Reduce the blender speed to the lowest and add the chia seeds.

3. Pour the content into an airtight container and put in a refrigerator for five to six hours.

4. To serve, you can garnish with the cinnamon powder of pomegranate seeds.

Nutrition: Calories: 201; Fat: 10 g; Sodium: 32.8 mg

42. Sweet Tahini Dip with Ginger Cinnamon Fruit

Preparation Time: 10 minutes

Cooking Time: 5 minutes

Servings: 2

Ingredients:

- Cinnamon, one (1) teaspoon
- Green apple, one (1)
- Pear, one (1)
- Fresh ginger, two (2) – three (3)
- Celtic sea salt, one (1) teaspoon
- Ingredient for sweet Tahini
- Almond butter (raw), three (3) teaspoons
- Tahini (one big scoop), three (3) teaspoons
- Coconut oil, two (2) teaspoons
- Cayenne (optional), ¼ teaspoons
- Wheat-free tamari, two (2) teaspoons
- Liquid coconut nectar, one (1) teaspoon

Directions:

1. Get a clean mixing bowl.
2. Grate the ginger, add cinnamon, sea salt and mix together in the bowl.
3. Dice apple and pear into little cubes, turn into the bowl and mix.
4. Get a mixing bowl and mix all the Ingredients.
5. Then add the Sprinkle the Sweet Tahini Dip all over the Ginger Cinnamon Fruit.
6. Serve.

Nutrition: Calories: 109; Fat: 10.8 g; Sodium: 258 mg

43. Coconut Butter and Chopped Berries with Mint

Preparation Time: 5 minutes
Cooking Time: 5 minutes
Servings: 4
Ingredients:

- Chopped mint, one (1) tablespoon
- Coconut butter (melted), two (2) tablespoons
- Mixed berries (strawberries, blueberries, and raspberries)

Directions:

1. Get a small bowl and add the berries.
2. Drizzle the melted coconut butter and sprinkle the mint.
3. Serve.

Nutrition: Calories: 159; Fat: 12 g; Carbohydrates: 18 g

Juice and Smoothie Recipes

44. Pineapple & Carrot Smoothie

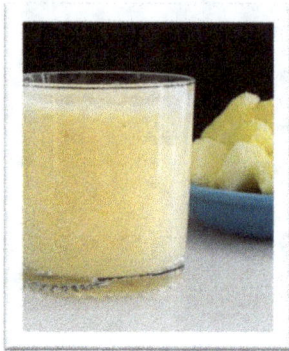

Preparation Time: 10 minutes
Cooking Time: 0 minutes
Servings: 2
Ingredients:

- 1 cup frozen pineapple
- 1 large ripe banana, peeled and sliced
- ½ tablespoon fresh ginger, peeled and chopped
- ¼ teaspoon ground turmeric
- 1 cup unsweetened almond milk
- ½ cup fresh carrot juice
- 1 tablespoon fresh lemon juice

Directions:

1. Place all the ingredients in a high-speed blender and pulse until creamy.

2. Pour the smoothie into two glasses and serve immediately.

Nutrition: Calories 132; Total Fat 2.2 g; Saturated Fat 0.3 g; Cholesterol 0 mg; Sodium 113 mg; Total Carbs 629.3 g; Fiber 4.1 g; Sugar 16.9 g; Protein 2 g;

45. Oats & Orange Smoothie

Preparation Time: 10 minutes

Cooking Time: 0 minutes

Servings: 4

Ingredients:

- 2/3 cup rolled oats
- 2 oranges, peeled, seeded, and sectioned
- 2 large bananas, peeled and sliced
- 2 cups unsweetened almond milk
- 1 cup ice cubes, crushed

Directions:

1. Place all the ingredients in a high-speed blender and pulse until creamy.
2. Pour the smoothie into four glasses and serve immediately.

Nutrition: Calories 175; Total Fat 3 g; Saturated Fat 0.4 g; Cholesterol 0 mg; Sodium 93 mg; Total Carbs 36.6 g; Fiber 5.9 g, Sugar 17.1 g, Protein 3.9 g;

46. Pumpkin Smoothie

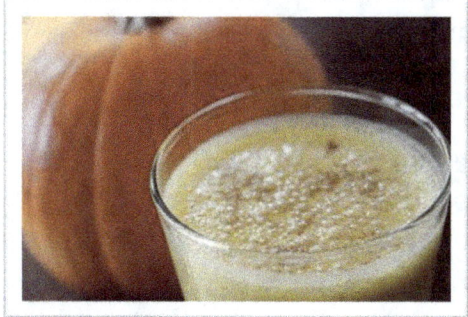

Preparation Time: 10 minutes

Cooking Time: 0 minutes

Servings: 2

Ingredients:

- 1 cup homemade pumpkin puree
- 1 medium banana, peeled and sliced
- 1 tablespoon maple syrup
- 1 teaspoon ground flaxseeds
- ½ teaspoon ground cinnamon
- ¼ teaspoon ground ginger
- 1½ cups unsweetened almond milk
- ¼ cup ice cubes

Directions:

1. Place all the ingredients in a high-speed blender and pulse until creamy.

2. Pour the smoothie into two glasses and serve immediately.

Nutrition: Calories 159; Total Fat 3.6 g; Saturated Fat 0.5 g; Cholesterol 0 mg; Sodium 143 mg; Total Carbs 32.6 g; Fiber 6.5 g, Sugar 17.3 g; Protein 3 g

47. Red Veggie & Fruit Smoothie

Preparation Time: 10 minutes
Cooking Time: 0 minutes
Servings: 2
Ingredients:

- ½ cup fresh raspberries
- ½ cup fresh strawberries
- ½ red bell pepper, seeded and chopped
- ½ cup red cabbage, chopped
- 1 small tomato
- 1 cup water
- ½ cup ice cubes

Directions:

1. Place all the ingredients in a high-speed blender and pulse until creamy.
2. Pour the smoothie into two glasses and serve immediately.

Nutrition: Calories 39; Cholesterol 0 mg; Saturated Fat 0 g; Sodium 10 mg; Total Carbs 8.9 g; Fiber 3.5 g; Sugar 4.8 g; Protein 1.3 g, Total Fat 0.4 g

48. Kale Smoothie

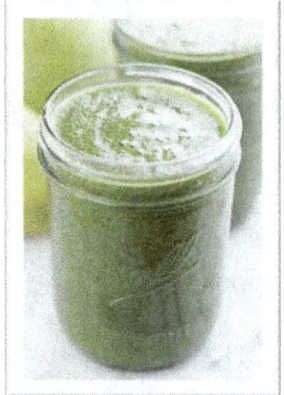

Preparation Time: 10 minutes
Cooking Time: 0 minutes
Servings: 2
Ingredients:

- 3 stalks fresh kale, trimmed and chopped
- 1-2 celery stalks, chopped
- ½ avocado, peeled, pitted, and chopped
- ½-inch piece ginger root, chopped
- ½-inch piece turmeric root, chopped
- 2 cups coconut milk

Directions:

1. Place all the ingredients in a high-speed blender and pulse until creamy.

2. Pour the smoothie into two glasses and serve immediately.

Nutrition: Calories 248; Total Fat 21.8 g; Saturated Fat 12 g; Cholesterol 0 mg; Sodium 59 mg; Total Carbs 11.3 g; Fiber 4.2 g; Sugar 0.5 g, Protein 3.5 g

Ù

49. Green Tofu Smoothie

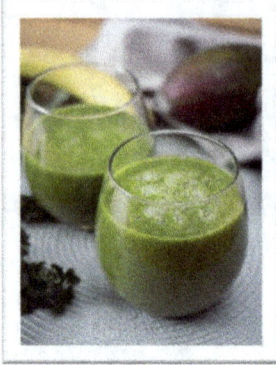

Preparation Time: 10 minutes

Cooking Time: 0 minutes

Servings: 2

Ingredients:

- 1½ cups cucumber, peeled and chopped roughly
- 3 cups fresh baby spinach
- 2 cups frozen broccoli
- ½ cup silken tofu, drained and pressed
- 1 tablespoon fresh lime juice
- 4-5 drops liquid stevia
- 1 cup unsweetened almond milk
- ½ cup ice, crushed

Directions:

1. Place all the ingredients in a high-speed blender and pulse until creamy.

2. Pour the smoothie into two glasses and serve immediately.

Nutrition: Calories 118; Total Fat 15 g; Saturated Fat 0.8 g; Cholesterol 0 mg; Sodium 165 mg; Total Carbs 12.6 g; Fiber 4.8 g; Sugar 3.4 g; Protein 10 g

50. Grape & Swiss Chard Smoothie

Preparation Time: 10 minutes

Cooking Time: 0 minutes

Servings: 2

Ingredients:

- 2 cups seedless green grapes
- 2 cups fresh Swiss chard, trimmed and chopped
- 2 tablespoons maple syrup
- 1 teaspoon fresh lemon juice
- 1½ cups water
- 4 ice cubes

Directions:

1. Place all the ingredients in a high-speed blender and pulse until creamy.
2. Pour the smoothie into two glasses and serve immediately.

Nutrition: Calories 176; Total Fat 0.2 g; Saturated Fat 0 g; Cholesterol 0 mg; Sodium 83 mg; Total Carbs 44.9 g; Fiber 1.7 g; Sugar 37.9 g; Protein 0.7 g

51. Matcha Smoothie

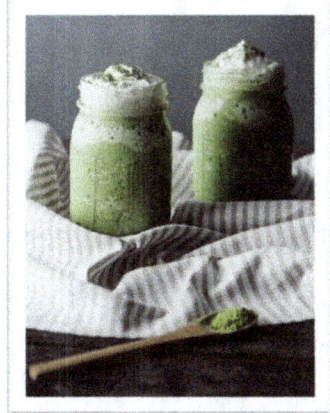

Preparation Time: 10 minutes
Cooking Time: 0 minutes
Servings: 2
Ingredients:

- 2 tablespoons chia seeds
- 2 teaspoons matcha green tea powder
- ½ teaspoon fresh lemon juice
- ½ teaspoon xanthan gum
- 8-10 drops liquid stevia
- 4 tablespoons coconut cream
- 1½ cups unsweetened almond milk
- ¼ cup ice cubes

Directions:
1. Place all the ingredients in a high-speed blender and pulse until creamy.
2. Pour the smoothie into two glasses and serve immediately.

Nutrition: Calories 132; Total Fat 12.3 g; Saturated Fat 6.8 g; Cholesterol 0 mg; Sodium 15 mg; Total Carbs 7 g; Fiber 4.8 g; Sugar 1 g; Protein 3 g

Conclusion

Being diagnosed with diabetes will bring about some major changes in your lifestyle. From the moment you are diagnosed, it will always be a constant battle with food. You have to become much more mindful of your food choices and the amount you eat. Every meal will feel like a major effort to you. You will plan each day throughout the week well in advance. Depending on the type of food you ate, you need to keep checking your blood sugar levels. You may get used to taking long breaks between meals and not snacking between dinner and breakfast. Managing diabetes can be a very, very stressful ordeal. There will be many times when you will mark your glucose levels on a piece of paper as if you are drawing graphic lines or something. You'll mix up your insulin shots and then you'll stress about whether you're giving yourself the right dosage. You will always be overly cautious because it's a lot of math and a very slim margin of error. But now, those days are over! The warning symptoms of type 1 diabetes are the same as in type 2; however, in type 1, these signs and symptoms tend to occur slowly over a period of months or years, making it more difficult to detect and recognize. Some of these symptoms may occur even after the disease has progressed. Diabetes can occur at any age. However, being too young or too old means your body is not in its best shape, and therefore, this increases your risk of developing diabetes.

Sounds scary. However, diabetes only occurs with the presence of a combination of these risk factors. Most risk factors can be minimized by taking action. For example, developing a more active lifestyle, taking care of your habits and trying to lower your blood sugar by limiting your sugar intake. If you start to notice that you are prediabetic or overweight, etc., there is always something you can do to change the situation. Recent studies show that developing healthy eating habits and following low carb diets, losing excess weight and leading an active lifestyle can help protect you from developing diabetes, especially type 2 diabetes, by minimizing the risk factors of developing the disorder.

www.ingramcontent.com/pod-product-compliance
Lightning Source LLC
Chambersburg PA
CBHW070932080526
44589CB00013B/1490